Oregano Oil

A Better Health Guide to Essential Oregano Oil Benefits, Uses, and Recipes

KARA AIMER

CONTENTS

INTRODUCTION

It is something that has been talked about everywhere from the *Dr. Oz Show* to *The View* to *Huffington Post*: Oregano Oil (or Oil of Oregano, as some call it). This so called "miracle cure" has been touted as one of the newest healing serums that will have you looking and feeling younger in a more healthier, easier way than some of the methods we have today. Even more, it has been called the future of the medical industry and the cure of the future.

Oil of Oregano has been declared a bit of a miracle for people within the beauty and health industry because even just a little dab on certain areas of the body yields results that are unprecedented. These capsules (or liquid, we'll discuss the merits of both later) work inside and outside of your body to help with problems that have no other cures or solutions. It will also take the place of some of the products that you have that either aren't very good for you or aren't very good for your wallet.

In this book, you will read about various ways to use oregano oil, methods to try, and even some recipes that will have you jumping up and running to your kitchen to try them out. It isn't difficult to make or use, and the oil will actually take the place of some of your current products.

You must first understand that everyone will have different results while using oil of oregano. You must also realize that everyone has a different timeline: Don't use oil of oregano for a single time and expect miracles. Instead, keep up with a routine that will last you a few weeks so that you can really see the improvements as they occur. You should also make sure that you are using a quality product: spending a little more on high-quality oregano oil will definitely help you here.

Of course, we all know about the joys of oregano in cooking, especially in Italian cooking, but what about the joys of oregano in other forms? You won't find the oregano we talk about in this book on the shelf in your local grocery store. Instead, the best results will come from the essential oil kind or the pill form. Though, you should also note that there are benefits to using more oregano in your cooking.

Read on to hear about the best things that can come from your use of oregano oil, and maybe even find a few solutions for problems that you thought you would always have to live with and never find relief for. More and more research is coming out about oregano oil, so keep your eyes and ears open to the benefits as there are probably going to be more released soon!

Congratulations on taking steps to living a fuller, better, healthier and more beautiful life with oregano oil!

WHAT IS OREGANO OIL

Oregano oil is a somewhat thick liquid that is derived from the leaves and the flowers of oregano or oreganum vulgare. This plant is hardy, bushy, and perennial, which means that the oil is one of the most inexpensive types of essential oils. Once again, that doesn't mean you should purchase the cheapest oregano oil that you find. It is actually a member of the mint family, which is why the taste is somewhat strong and the odor is distinct. Oregano is native to Europe but has been successfully cultivated all over the world and in many different climates. Originally, the plant wasn't used for spices and cooking like it is today.

The Greeks and Romans used the plant for medicinal purposes and healing but found that they did not hate the taste of it when consumed in broths or teas. The name "oregano" comes from the Greek word "oros" (mountain) and the word "ganos" (joy), which means that together, oregano is "the joy of the mountain." Over time, the herb has also been used as a symbol of happiness and celebration, often being included in crowns for royal inaugurations and bridal parties. As civilization grew, more and more strains and species of oregano came to life.

But oregano isn't just one type of plant – there are actually well over 40 species known to humans, though some of them aren't as good for healing as others are. The most therapeutic, and the one sold the most often, is the oil produced from origanum vulgare, or the wild oregano that is found throughout the Mediterranean basin. Be sure that if you are using oregano oil, it comes from oregano based in that area. Most grocery store types will come from the United States, and therefore, won't have the same results. Spain also has a species, thymus capitatus, which is great medicinally as well. To obtain oregano oil, the dried flowers and leaves of the wild oregano plant are harvested when the oil content of the plant is at its highest, and then distilled.

When purchasing, you want your oregano oil to have a dark yellow color and a very strong, spicy odor. Typically, you should also look for a container that is darker and stored in a dark part of the store.

COMPOSITION

Many people like to know about the composition of oregano oil, especially because they will be putting it onto their skin, which goes into their bloodstream. Oregano oil is extremely high in something called phenols, which is a natural compound that has antioxidant effects. Thymol, one of those phenols, is a natural fungicide with antiseptic qualities. It works to boost the immune system while shielding against tissue damage. Another phenol, carvacrol, helps your body fight off infections like candida albicans, staphylococcus, E. coli, campylobacter, salmonella, klebsiella, the aspergillus mold, giardia, pseudomonas, and listeria.

There are other phenols found in oregano oil that help with your body's healing and functioning as well. They include terpenes, which have antibacterial properties, rosmarinic acid, which is a powerful antioxidant that prevents free radical damage, helps against allergies and asthma and even has been shown to prevent cancer. Rosmarinic acid also reduces fluid buildup in the body. Finally, naringin stops the growth of cancer cells.

Some types of oregano also contain Beta-caryophyllin (E-BCP) which is often recommended for people with osteoporosis, arteriosclerosis, and metabolic problems.

Of course, the oil also contains more common nutrients as well, such as vitamins A, C, and E, magnesium, potassium, iron, calcium, manganese, boron, niacin, and copper.

Oregano oil is one of the most widespread medicines used in non-western medicine. We will talk more about the health and beautiful benefits in detail in a later chapter. However, it is best to note that even when you are working on something else within your body, you will still get these benefits..

BENEFITS OF OREGANO OIL

So we've already started going over some of the benefits of using oregano oil in your daily life – but that is just what it is, a start. There are plenty of benefits of using oregano oil, including benefits we haven't even discovered yet.

Everything in health and beauty starts with the inside of your body – how you feel and how your body works have a great impact on your general mood and daily life, even if you think you already feel fine. Many people don't realize just how lousy they actually feel until they start feeling better: and then they reap the benefits when they start to feel better. Using just a bit of oregano oil will make you feel better. As we chronicled in the last chapter, oregano oil is full of healthy vitamins and antioxidants that will encourage overall health and wellness. It will encourage your body functions to perform like a well-oiled machine, and will leave you feeling livelier.

But beyond those antioxidants and vitamins, oregano has other far-reaching health benefits that are more specific and targeted. Mostly, it has been linked to helping with respiratory and immune system wellness. The treatment of these problems includes preventing and treating infections of the body. The most common infection oregano oil treats is urinary tract infections or UTIs that are caused by bacteria that gets into our bodies, bacteria like E. coli, Proteus, and Pseudomonas aeruginosa. It also helps to clear up yeast infections (often confused with UTIs), especially in people who are resistant to other types of antifungal medications.

Moving up the body, oil of oregano treats respiratory infections caused by the Klebsiella pneumoniae and Staphylococcus aureus bacteria strains. It also helps to treat (in conjunction with other medications) parasitic infections that are caused by the amoeba giardia. Some people even have found that it works alone to treat some of these problems, but that hasn't been proven in all people yet.

Finally, oil of oregano has been shown to help fight off the deadly infection that can cause loss of limbs or blood infection, methicillin-resistant staphylococcus aureus infections, better known as MRSA.

OTHER BENEFITS

Oregano oil isn't only good for the inside of your body, however. It has also been found to help with a wide range of problems that plague humans. Oregano oil is currently being studied to see if it helps to prevent food borne illnesses that are caused by pathogens like listeria, salmonella, E. coli, and Shigella dysenteria. It is added to the food to help keep bacteria levels low, and will also alleviate food poisoning if the food isn't cooked properly. One study, out of the University of Arizona, has also found that oil of oregano can actually help to kill the norovirus, which is what causes uncomfortable stomach cramping and diarrhea.

AROMATHERAPHY

Since oregano oil is an essential oil, many have found other uses for it through steaming. Using an appropriate oil steamer, not just a wax heater, which is available from most health stores, the phenols can be released into the air and give a pleasant smell that is also healing. The steam method may help with some of the problems above, especially to reduce congestion and eliminate nausea, there are many other benefits with steaming.

The scent will actually ward off insects both inside and outside. If you don't want to use a steamer on your back porch, you can put a few drops on your outdoor furniture or make your own natural insect repellant by mixing some of the oil with water and putting it onto your skin. This works because of the carvacrol in the natural oil, which insects do not like the smell nor the taste of.

If it is too late and you've already been bitten by the bugs, or you have some kind of rash, including contact dermatitis or poison ivy, you can use the oregano oil to help reduce the swelling, redness, and itchiness. Use a mixture of oregano oil that has been diluted with olive oil and apply to the affected areas. This mixture may also help to prevent any scarring.

In addition to preventing scarring from rashes and hives, there are some other skin conditions that you will find oregano oil helps. Cold sores and pimples will shrink down and dry up with just a touch of oregano oil, dandruff will disappear if you use oregano oil once every two washes, and rosacea will clear up and stay away with just a little bit applied with lotion.

If you have a sore throat, especially on those spring mornings when you wake up and allergies have taken over, simply put a few drops of oregano oil into a glass of water (it doesn't mix well with orange juice) and drink it down. The oregano oil with soothe your throat. It will also do the same thing for toothaches, but the effect won't last quite as long.

Many personal trainers and those in physical therapy also use oil of oregano to help with the pain from sprains, pulls, twists, and breaks. Even some big name athletes have praised oregano oil, from football players and baseball players to gymnasts and figure skaters.

Finally, many people, especially older people who have tried everything else, have found that oregano oil, whether rubbed directly onto the skin or absorbed through pills and steam, will reduce the effects and aid with movement in those suffering from joint pain, muscle weakness or rheumatoid arthritis.

Keep in mind that the benefits of oregano oil are vast, and we do not even understand all of its power yet. Scientists are still studying and learning about this "miracle" oil.

If you are interested in finding out about more of the cures and treatments mentioned above, a later chapter will go into further detail about how to fix some of those problems and many more.

SIDE EFFECTS

As with any type of medication, whether it is natural or prescription, oil of oregano will have some type of side effects that might void out some of the benefits for users. However, the side effects with oregano oil are often mild, and most of the time won't even show up in otherwise healthy individuals. However, it is still best to know about them so that you can weigh your pros and cons:

Feeling

If you apply lotion as a topical, you might feel a few different things. First, your skin may tingle or feel greasy. This is just a part of using any type of lotion, and that feeling will actually start to feel good: it is why so many athletes and physical therapists use it for injuries.

Some people, especially those who use oregano oil or rashes, hives, or bug bites, have said that they experience more tingling, and some even experience a burning sensation when they first use the product. This can be attributed, more often, to the lotions that you mix the product with for application.

Taste

Taking oregano oil capsules is much like taking any other type of medication. You will be able to taste the pill a little bit, but you typically will only feel it going down your throat. However, the pills do dissolve quickly and you should take care to not cut or squish the pills, and then you might get the strong taste in your mouth.

There have been very few reports of indigestion or burping of the oil back up that people typically experience with fish oils.

The oil of oregano that you make yourself might have a stronger taste than the type you buy the in store – that is just a byproduct of making it by yourself. It will also depend on the type of carrier oil (more on that later) that you use with the oil.

Length
The length of time that someone can take oil of oregano has not truly been studied. However, because it is all natural, there seems to be a limitless time. You should take great care to feel out your body and see if the product is still working for you. You might have to play around with levels and density of the product after a few uses, especially if you are in a lot of pain.

However, if you are using oregano oil for health benefits that impact your daily life, you might want to use them for about a month before going to the doctor or dentist to have it looked over by a professional – no matter how you feel.

Physical
As always, some of the more nutritional foods might do some pretty unexpected things to your body, especially if you aren't used to eating healthy foods. Some people, especially those who have sensitive stomachs, may experience nausea and stomach upset when ingesting oregano oil or the herb. Typically, these people have a better result when they consume the tablet form, but not always. Those who are allergic to plants from the Lamiaceae family, especially mint, lavender, sage, and basil, should also avoid this oil, as they may also develop an allergic reaction.

Any other allergy problems, including gluten and dairy problems, should not have any problem with taking an oregano supplement or oregano oil. Just make sure to double check the ingredients, especially if you take the tablet. Usually, you can avoid this if you buy higher quality oregano oil.

Once again, this is most easily avoided if you make your own oil of oregano instead of purchasing it from the store.

.

DO NOT TAKE

Oregano oil is also NOT advisable for infants, children, and anyone under the age of 15. This is mostly because of body functions that are still developing, but that depends on the person. If you think your child or teen would benefit, you should talk to his or her doctor.

Pregnant or nursing women should also ask their doctors if it is okay to use. Generally, however, the use of oregano oil by pregnant and nursing women is discouraged because it can encourage the blood circulation that happens around and within the uterus, which can actually deteriorate the lining that encompasses the fetus within the womb, which can have some negative effects on the fetus and the birthing process. Oregano oil also has a potential to induce menstruation by thinning out the mucus lining of your uterus, and could be dangerous if you are carrying a child.

People who are very sick and undergoing cancer treatments should also check with their doctor before taking oil of oregano, just to make sure that it won't interact with any of the medicine you are currently using.

MAKE YOUR OWN

Some people, especially those who don't like to put preservatives into their bodies, like to make their own supplements. While it is possible to buy the essential oil in its purest form, some people just like the process of making their own. Making your own oil of oregano can be somewhat difficult the first few times, but is fairly simple for those who have done it for a few months.

This is just one method, and there are a few on the internet and in other books. However, these steps work best for beginners and those who don't plan to mass produce oil of oregano for bottling.

The ratio for making oil of oregano is actually pretty simple: 1:1. The biggest thing you will need is patience, as it will take at least two weeks for your first batch to be ready for use.

You will use half a cup of oil and a half a cup of dried and chopped oregano leaves. If you use fresh oregano, it will have to be completely devoid of any excess water, or you will face problems. Fresh oregano also has a higher rate of going rancid and developing mold.

For the oil, you can use any kind of oil you prefer, but most people suggest using olive oil, almond oil, or grape seed oil. Some people have successfully used coconut oil, but others haven't had great results.

This method will take a while, so remember that you need to have patience.

How to Make Your Own Oil of Oregano

Step 1: Get some filtered, clean water and bring it to a rolling boil in a sauce pan. Let it boil for about three minutes before completely turning off the heat – you can let the water sit on the saucepan. You will need at least a few cups of water.

Step 2: Sanitize a mason or other glass jar so that it is completely void of any bacteria or dust. A bottle sanitizer would work well here.

Step 3: Place your oil of choice in the jar, filling it until it is a little less than halfway full. Then, you should put in the oregano leaves until the jar is filled. Place a lid firmly on the jar.

Step 4: Place the jar into the hot water on your stove and allow it to sit for at least ten minutes. This process allows the oil to heat up and helps to give the oregano a start to the chemical process that it needs to release any of the oils it has in the leaves. You should be able to see the oils start to leave and infiltrate the oil.

Step 5: Remove the jar from the water and completely dry it, making sure to be extra through along the rim and around the lid of the jar – you want to completely remove any water so there isn't any mold or growth.

Step 6: Find the sunniest window in your house – or the window that receives the most constant sunlight – and let it sit for 1-2 weeks. If you wish, you can move the jar from window to window as the day passes and the sun moves. This will speed up the process so that you can get started sooner.

Step 7: Every few days, you will want to shake the jar and then twist it in a figure eight pattern. This will help to stop the separation that naturally occurs between the oil and what the leaves excrete. Avoid doing this every day, as you will cause the leaves to break down unnaturally.

Step 8: Once you see no more movement or deterioration of the leaves for a few days, or once the two weeks is up, you can open up the jar. You should take a strainer and try to remove all of the leaves from the oil. Strain into another sanitized jar. You do not want to use the same jar, and you don't want to strain into something else and then put it back into the original jar. Strain right into a new sanitized jar.

Step 9: Store the oil in a kitchen or bathroom cabinet that is dark and hidden from the light. You do not want to put the jar near anything that gets too warm or too cool. You should also try to keep any condensation away from the jar, as that can contaminate it.

Tips:
Take great care to not infect the lip or inside of the jar when you use the oil. Your best choice will be to pour just a little bit of the oil onto your hand. You might get some of the oil on the outside of the jar, but you can just wipe that down. Sticking anything inside of the jar will create an unstable environment.

Some people have said that putting a drop or two of grape seed oil inside of the jar when you use it will help to kill off any bacteria that are growing inside.

You should also make sure to look at the quality and state of your homemade oil when you use your jar. Hold it up to the light and make sure it isn't too cloudy or clumpy. If you notice that the texture, appearance, or smell of the oil is off, you will want to throw the oil away.

HEALTH BENEFITS

The health benefits of oil or oregano make it one of the most diverse items in your medicine cabinet. Try to always keep some on hand, as you don't know when you will need it!

Throughout this section and the next section, we will talk about mixing oregano oil with carrier oils. A carrier oil is a completely vegan oil that is typically from the fatty portion of a plant, most likely from seeds, kernels, and/or nuts. Do not apply carrier oils by themselves, as they can actually cause rashes and dryness if they serve no purpose. Some of the cures will call for specific oil, but most will just call for a carrier oil of your choice. The most commonly used oil is coconut oil.

Carrier oils include: Almond Oil, Apricot Kernel Oil, Avocado Oil, Borage Oil, Calendula Oil, Cocoa Butter, Coconut Oil, Evening Primrose Oil, Grapeseed Oil, Hazelnut Oil, Jojoba Oil, Kukui Oil, Macadamia Nut Oil, Olive Oil, Peanut Oil, Pecan Oil, Rose Hip Oil, Sesame Oil, Shea Butter, Sunflower Oil, Walnut Oil, and Wheat germ Oil.

Here are just a few of the most common uses of oregano oil for health:

Capsules
A note about oil of oregano capsules: if something on this list is to

be done topically, you might get the same results by taking daily oil of oregano capsules. You also might not, especially if your situation is extremely bad.

Sanitizer
To make a natural hand sanitizer that won't dry or hurt your hands, simply combine about ten drops of oregano oil (essential of what you just made) with two tablespoons of coconut oil. From there, you will be able to rub it in as a natural, moisturizing hand sanitizer.

House Cleaning Tools
Add a few drops to a half of a cup (depending on what you are cleaning and how much) of oregano oil to your cleaning supplies to give them an antiseptic and disinfectant boost. This will work best in the cleaning supplies that you make yourself. If you wish to combine with store bought cleaning supplies, mix in a separate container than the one you store the cleaner in. This method is especially effective in the kitchen and in the bathroom, where the most germs are.

Toothpaste
For an all-natural toothpaste, simply use a few drops of oil of oregano on your toothbrush. If you want a whitening toothpaste, you can mix the oil with baking soda on your toothbrush. If you don't like the feeling of the oil in your mouth (which many don't), you should follow with a mouthwash. You can use the following mouthwash:

Mouthwash
Add a few drops to a glass of water to sweeten your breath and kill the bacteria that can lead to gum disease and gingivitis.

Ringworm
To kill ringworm, only on humans, not animals, apply 3 to 6 drops of non-diluted oregano oil to the affected area. Do this a few times a day until the symptoms go away.

Colds
If you have a cold that just won't quit, or you can't stand having a stuffy nose, oregano oil can help. Simply put some oil of oregano

(essential oils or the oil you made above) into a diffuser and allow it to circulate throughout the night. You should feel better after a few hours. This won't cure the cold, but it will stop the symptoms.

You could also use oregano oil to steam open your nasal passages. Simply put some oil of oregano into a pot, heat the water, and inhale the steam. Make sure not to burn your skin, and only do this for a few minutes. You can also use the oil like a vapor rub and put it just under your nostrils to help you breath more easily.

Sore Throats
To ease the pain, scratchiness, and even the loss of your voice that comes with a sore throat, simply add one or two drops of oregano essential oil to a glass of water of juice and drink it down. Once again, this won't cure your sore throat, but it will allow you to feel better.

Intestinal Problems
Oil of oregano works to keep your intestines healthy and clean. You will find yourself more "regular" and that it won't hurt to go to the bathroom. It will also help to clear your intestines of bacteria, which is especially a problem in people who are spending a great deal of time in the hospital.

Athlete's Foot
To reduce the itching and burning that occurs with athlete's foot, especially at night, dilute oil of oregano into a carrier oil and apply directly as needed, up to five times a day, and then immediately cover with thick socks. You can also add a few drops to baking soda to sprinkle inside your shoes for added protection.

Arthritis
To stop the pain that is associated with an arthritic flare, dilute oregano oil and rub onto painful joints to decrease the swelling. This will also work with any sports injuries.

Anti-Fungal
Oil of oregano is a great antifungal because it does not allow the fungus to develop a resistance. Oil of oregano is one of the best cures for yeast infections because of this, as a woman who has a

yeast infection often develops resistance to the antibiotics.

Insect Repellent

To make a natural insect repellant that won't make you smell like a day old vodka bottle, simply mix a few drops of oregano oil into a salve or carrier oil and rub it into your skin, focusing on your pulse points. If you want to plan ahead, you can also mix the oil with half oregano oil and water to make your own repellant. If you put it into a spray jar, just make sure you shake well before spraying.

Bug Bites

If you already have bug bites, a rash, or hives from something in the environment, you can use a salve of oregano oil mixed with lotion or topical ointments and allowing it to dry. Many people recommend putting a drop of the oregano oil on the spot right before bed, and then using a Band-Aid to keep it against the skin.

Psoriasis

To ward off a psoriasis outbreak, mix oil of oregano with a salve or carrier oil. You should do this once in the morning and once at night. If you don't want to rub it into your skin (if you are too sensitive) you can also try to drink a glass of water twice a day that has 2-6 drops of oregano oil mixed into it.

Eczema

Control eczema outbreaks, dryness, or bleeding by blending oregano oil with carrier oil or salve and applying topically to the infected area. Some even say that you can use this when you feel an outbreak coming.

Diaper Rash and Chafing

If you have talked to your doctor and he or she thinks it is okay to use oregano oil on your baby, you can use a combination of coconut oil and oregano oil to soothe and heal any diaper rash. It will also work for chafing that occurs under the arms, on the genitals, or between the legs.

BEAUTY BENEFITS

It has been said that everything we need on earth to survive and to thrive has been provided for us. That's why some people find it crazy that people will spend $200 on a single jar of face cream or over $1,000 for surgeries to make things look better.

Oregano oil is one of the cures for many of today's beauty ailments. Even if you wouldn't classify your problem as an ailment, using oil of oregano as part of your daily beauty regimen may help you.

SPOT TREATMENT

If you have a lot of acnes or you have dark marks and scars from previous bouts of acne, you can use oregano oil to help you clear up your skin for good. Simple dip a cotton swab into the oil and put a drop or two on the pimple, boil, or mark. Leave it on, especially overnight, and you will see an instant reaction. The oil will not only eliminate redness and swelling, it will also kill the bacteria, shortening the life of the pimple. For the best results, do this after you wash your face at night and allow it to sit on your face while you sleep. You can also do it in the morning for a shorter time for smaller pimples or areas of redness. If you apply this paste to other parts of your body, make sure to keep it out of any mucus membranes.

If you have a skin infection, dilute some oil of oregano into coconut oil and apply onto your skin to clear up the infection. This will also work for breakouts.

Warts and Skin Tags
Warts and skin tags aren't always the most attractive things in the world, but they are also harmless. However, if they do bother you, oregano oil can help you. Simply apply one or two drops of oregano oil onto the infected area in the morning and cover with a Band-Aid to keep it on. Then, apply another drop at night that you keep open to the air. If you do this every day, the warts will start to dry up. Your skin tags will also dry up and then fall off.

Some people also recommend mixing together coconut oil and oregano oil so that it stays on more, especially if you have the problem at a place where a Band Aid won't stay on throughout the day.

Dandruff

Dandruff, or dry skin on your head, can also be cured by oil of oregano. Simply take your favorite shampoo and mix a few drops into the bottle. Many people will keep a small bottle in their bathroom to add it right into the product on their hand. This is especially recommended for severe cases. Just make sure to keep your shampoo out of your eyes, as the oregano oil will definitely burn.

Make sure to add this to your shampoo and not your conditioner, or it will not work as well. You can also use oil or oregano in a hot oil treatment to make your hair healthier – simply mix a few drops into your treatment.

Bleeding Gums

Bleeding gums are often a sign that you aren't paying as much attention to your oral hygiene as you should. If this isn't the case and your gums are still bleeding, you may need to take action. Combine a drop or two of oregano oil with one drop of a carrier oil, coconut oil is suggested. Do something called "oil pulling" or swishing the substance around like you would with a mouthwash. Do NOT spit this into your sink. Instead, spit it into a tissue and throw away – you will clog your pipes if you don't.

This can be a part of a full oral routine that you use with oregano oil. After doing this for a few weeks, you might want to go to your dentist, who will tell you if your new routine is successful.

Laundry

Many people are now looking for more environmentally friendly ways to do their laundry. A great way to do this while still getting everything clean is to add a few drops of oregano oil to your load of laundry to kill the bacteria or parasites. Your clothes will still smell great and will actually hold their scent for a longer amount of time.

If you have more expensive clothes, you should add a few drops to your bleach dispenser, which will disperse the oil and not risk your clothing.

Cold Sores

If you have painful cold sores on your lip, you can use oregano oil to stop the pain, erase the redness, and cure them faster. Simply put a drop or two directly on the mark. You can do this before or after any other ointments you put on your skin.

Some people also say that oil of oregano will work on canker sores, but there has been a very little study into that.

Nail Fungus

If you have dry, cracked, or bubbling nails, oregano might be able to help. Soak your hands or your feet in a basin of warm water and Epsom salt with a few teaspoons of oregano oil added in before your feet even touch the water. You can also add some essential oils to help with the smell, if you wish. Allow your feet to soak for 10-15 minutes or until the water is cold. When you are finished soaking your feet, rub diluted oil (1 drop of oil in a teaspoon of carrier oil) directly onto your nails. You can do the same thing for your hands, if you wish.

Note that oregano oil is also great for softening your cuticles and nailbeds.

ANTIBIOTICS

When doctors developed antibiotics, they thought they had found the answer to many of today's health problems and infections. However, what they didn't expect is that we would develop immunities to these pills, and we would have to look elsewhere. Oregano oil is one of those places that scientists, doctors, and healers alike now look for a new cure or treatment.

Oregano oil doesn't cause some of the side effects, like reduced vitamin absorption, deterioration of good bacteria, and leaky gut. Many people are now turning to oregano oil, even if they aren't resistant to the pills. Oil of oregano contains two powerful compounds that we have already talked about: carvacrol and thymol. They both have powerful anti-bacterial and anti-fungal properties.

Many different people have done research on the use of oregano oil versus the use of prescription antibiotics, and the results have been staggering. They found that nearly 60% of the people who used antibiotics would have benefitted from oregano in the same way.

While this might not seem like a problem, remember that the more a person uses antibiotics, the less effective they are. By using oil of oregano for the problem, you are saving yourself for a time when you really need them.

To date, there have been over 800 studies that looked at oil of oregano, and they have found that it is effective in treating: Bacterial infections, fungal infections, parasites, viruses, inflammation, candida, allergies, and tumors.

The Journal of Medicinal Food recently published a study that showed that using oil of oregano as an antibacterial aid makes your body resistant against five different types of bad bacteria that can make us sick. These types are the most common form of bacteria that make us sick, cause us to feel lethargic, and that infiltrate into our homes.

The bad bacteria that it works the best against is actually the deadly E. Coli, which is the leading cause of gastrointestinal problems and food poisoning. Earlier in this book, you read about using oregano oil in your cleaning supplies and to clean out your intestines. While there hasn't been a long-term study into the effectiveness, the oil has been used outside of western medicine for some time.

Interestingly, a team of researchers in Pakistan have actually claimed that they have used oregano oil to kill cancer cells and that it might be the answer to some of our most complicated types of cancer.

Of course, remember that it is never a good idea to self-diagnose or self-treat. If you have a problem, you should talk to your doctor or dentist about the best way to proceed. Typically, you doctor will recommend a more medicinal path, but won't dissuade you from using oil of oregano.

CONCLUSION

By now, you have probably come to understand that the herb that you keep in your kitchen cabinets is probably one of the most beneficial things you can keep in your house. While it isn't the "cure all" that many people are looking for, it is definitely a "cure most" for many people.

The best way to start using oil of oregano, especially if this is your first time venturing into natural cures, is to just listen to your body. Your body will tell you if things are working, or if maybe that particular healing method doesn't work for you. Remember that every single person is different, and that if you have something different in your health history, a different lifestyle, or even just a different heritage, you may have a completely different reaction to the use of oil of oregano.

The best thing to do is to start with just a little bit of oil of oregano that you purchase from your local health store. You might start using it as a toothpaste, a topical ointment, or a nail treatment before you start using it to treat other problems.

Only once you recognize how you feel using the oil of oregano will you be able to make your own. Compare how you feel with your handmade oil and how you felt with the store bought oil.

It is a process, and you might not always be able to figure out how or if the oil is working. However, you should stick with the process for more than just a few days to see if it is worthwhile.

Good luck, and congratulations on starting your path toward a happier, healthier, and more wholesome you!
Thank you and good luck!

Kara Aimer

ADDITIONAL RESOURCES

Please point your web browser to **www.plaid-enterprises.com**
for more related resources, my full bibliography and to grab your
FREE book!

www.ingramcontent.com/pod-product-compliance
Lightning Source LLC
Chambersburg PA
CBHW070935290526
45795CB00003B/1030